Fad Dieting

What you need to know...

http://www.diabetagon.com

Copyright © 2008 Nick Jakotic

Author: Nick Jakotic
Edition: 1st Edition
Printed by: Split Whisker Publishing
ISBN: 978-0-9805133-0-1
Dewey Number: 613.25
CiP: 14282

Table of Contents

Chapter 1 – What is a diet?

A diet actually refers to the type of foods that you eat. But a diet seems to mean something different to each individual. To some a diet is just simply eating healthy food choices while keeping unhealthy choices to a minimum. This does not fall into what a lot would call dieting but it is still a diet.

To others though, a diet is the latest fad on the market that promises to allow the individual to lose weight. This can take place in the form of diet drinks, limited food choices, pills and any other form that wishes to be used to promote weight loss. The question is do these dieting methods work and are these methods safe?

Fad diets have found themselves becoming more and more as dieters are seeking out the perfect way to lose weight. There is a reason they are referred to as a fad diet. Fads changes constantly and these diets will try to change to meet the latest fad that society is mostly following. Fads are not usually long term and most fad diets can not give you long term results.

Chapter 2 – The Food Pyramid is not a One Size Fits All

For decades the food pyramid was promoted to give a guideline to healthy eating. The food pyramid listed each category of foods that a person needed to eat daily to keep in good shape and be healthy. The problem is that when one does live by the food pyramid and still gains an unhealthy amount of weight. This left it to be questioned as to what was wrong with the food pyramid. The food pyramid was rewritten and a new pyramid was designed. This pyramid failed as a one size fits all pyramid just like the old pyramid had failed.

The latest development with the food pyramid was to realize that while everyone does need almost each and every category of food that is one the pyramid, not everyone needs the same amounts of those food.

Factors such as age, height, current weight and level of activity needed to be taken into consideration. Low and behold and new food pyramid was developed to allow for everyone to reach their ideal weight and maintain that weight.

The food pyramid website mypyramid.gov allows for you to enter the determining factors so that it can give you a food pyramid designed just for you. No more trying to eat from a pyramid that is designed for someone else's body type. This new pyramid will not only tell you how much you as an individual need to consume of each thing daily but also how much you need to work in of certain foods on a weekly basis.

Chapter 3 – The South Beach Diet

The South Beach diet was designed by an established cardiologist, Dr. Arthur Agatston around the mid 1990s. He created the diet based off his disbelief that the diet recommend by the American Heart Association worked in terms of long term results.

The South Beach diet is broken down into down into three phases that a you will work yourself through. Phase 1 is a two week phase in which you will cut out foods that contain carbohydrates, are loaded with sugar and you will also cut out alcohol. Phase 2 is the phase that you will begin at the end of two weeks. You will stay in this phase for as long as it take you to reach your ideal healthy weight. During this phase you will start adding back foods that you had removed during your phase 1 of your South Beach diet. You will be allowed to introduce wine at this phase and you will slowly introduce the right carbohydrates into you meals. Phase 3 is where you will continue to eat the food choices that you were taught during phase 1 and phase 2 for life. This phase was meant serve as a maintaining phase to help you maintain your new healthy weight indefinitely.

The South Beach diet book and website offer up recipes for each phase that can help you to create meals that fit with the phase you are in. It is designed to not only show you a new way to eat but also to help you learn how to fix these new foods.

Chapter 4 – Pros and Cons of the South Beach Diet

By weighing the pros and cons of the South Beach diet, you can better determine if this diet is right for you. When looking at the pros and cons you need to look at whether or not the weighing of the pros and cons will fit with your lifestyle as well. While the pros may out weight the cons, the diet still may or may not fit with your individual lifestyle. Ask yourself if this diet is something that you can stick with over the long term to see and maintain positive results.

The pros of the South Beach Diet:

- The diet works in stages to help you make changing in the way you eat.

- The giving up of foods is only for a short two weeks.
- The diet offers a lot of food choices that other diets may limit.
- There are no counting of carbohydrates or calories.
- The diet offers up recipes that will help you to know what to create with the foods you are allowed to eat.
- The diet will work you back up to eating most the foods that you may love.
- It is easy to eat out at restaurants with this diet.
- The diet is geared for a long term eating habit to help you maintain your ideal weight.

The cons of the South Beach Diet:

- Two weeks of giving up foods that you may be use to eating on a daily basis.

- Food list is seen by some as too restrictive.

- Going for two weeks with no carbohydrates and fats and then reintroducing them back in may cause you to feel slightly ill.

- The lack of structure when it comes to carbohydrates and fats. This leaves too much up to the individual and may result in diet failure.

- The diet uses a glycemic index that is not officially incorporated into dietary recommendations by the American Diabetes Association.

- Your body may go into ketosis while completely off carbohydrates for two weeks. Ketosis cause strain on the kidneys.

- There is not enough research to show what the long term effects of ketosis may have on the body.

Chapter 5 – The Atkins Diet

The Atkins diet was created by Dr. Robert Atkins originally in the 1960 and came back into focus in the 1990s. The diet is one that consists of high protein and low carbohydrate eating. With the Atkins diet a person can eat foods containing all the calories that they want the come from protein and fat. They must however restrict their carbohydrate intake.

In the most recent revisions of his book Dr. Atkins had address some misconception about his diet plan. One misconception is that you can consume all the fatty foods that you want. While the diet places no limit on the amount you can consume it does not give the go ahead for pigging out on junk foods or stuffing one's self full at meals.

The Atkins diet consists of four phases that you will work through while on the diet. Phase 1 is called the induction phase and is the phase that is the most restrictive in what you are allowed to eat. You will stay in phase 1 until you hit what is known as ketosis, which is usually 2 weeks. The second phase is known as the ongoing weight loss phase. During this phase you may increase your carbohydrate intake by 2 net grams each week. This phase will last until you are within 10 pounds of your desired weight. Phase 3 is the Pre-maintenance phase. During this phase you will increase your carbohydrate intake again and this time it will increase by 10 net carbohydrates. a week. You will stay in this phase until you find the amount of carbohydrate you can consume without gaining any weight. The last phase is the lifetime maintenance phase. This is where you will continue to eat the Atkins way for life.

The Atkins diet offers up health bars and shakes for those on the diet. As well a lot of restaurants are offering up dishes that conform to the Atkins diet approach. This allows for quick meals on the go, as well as the opportunity to eat out once in awhile and never stop your diet.

Chapter 6 - The Pros and Cons of the Atkins Diet

By weighing the pros and cons of the Atkins diet, you can better determine if this diet is right for you. When looking at the pros and cons you need to look at whether or not the weighing of the pros and cons will fit with your lifestyle as well. Not all diets are created equal when it comes to weight loss. This is where you need to really examine the pros and cons of a diet as well as finding your own pros and cons. This will let you know if the diet is right for you as an individual.

The pros of the Atkins diet:

- The diet allows for the steaks and hamburgers as regular menu items. This makes it more appealing to men.
- Research has shown that an Atkins dieter can lose lots of weight while on this diet.
- Cholesterol levels have been known to initially improve for dieters following the Atkins diet.
- There is no need for you to count calories while on the Atkins diet.

The cons of the Atkins diet:

- The foods allowed on the diet are very restrictive through out all phases of the diet.
- While you do not have to count calories while on the diet you must count carbohydrates while on the diet.
- The diet forces the body into ketosis. Ketosis causes strain on the kidneys and there does not seem to be enough research done yet to determine what long term effects ketosis may cause.
- Calcium levels are negatively effected on the Atkins diet.
- Once your weight has stabilized while on the Atkins diet, cholesterol levels may rise.

- Complications such as constipation and dehydration can occur while on the Atkins diet.

- Rare complications such as an increase risk of heart disease, hypertension and liver and kidney trouble are known to happen when on the Atkins diet.

Chapter 7 – Comparing the South Beach Diet and the Atkins Diet

While the South Beach diet and the Atkins diet differ in some ways from each other, there are of course similarities in the way that the diets work. Comparing these diets from each other can be done by looking at the similarities that the diets have in common as well as the looking at the differences between the two diets. This chapter is going to show you the similarities and the differences between the two diets.

The similarities between the South Beach diet and the Atkins diet:

The South Beach diet and the Atkins diet were both created by doctors. These doctors questioned the normal views on food against their own beliefs when creating their diets.

Both diets focus on limiting carbohydrates. With the belief that carbohydrates are what makes a person gain weight.

Neither diet has you counting calories or fat grams when you are on the diet. Both however do focus on the limiting of carbohydrates.

Both diets offer up recipes to help you when preparing foods appropriate with their diets.

You can actually eat out while on both of these diets without going off the diet. The

Atkins diet actual appears on many menus in restaurants.

The South Beach diet and the Atkins diet offer foods that you can purchase.

Both diets have been known to cause a danger reaction in the body known as ketosis.

Both diets have come under criticism from the medical community.

Both diets have books written by the creators and websites put together to help you with your dieting.

Now that we have looked at the similarities between both the South Beach diet and the Atkins diet, let us now take a look at how these diets differ.

The differences between the South Beach diet and the Atkins diet:

The South Beach diet focuses on removing all carbohydrates during the first two weeks then reintroducing good carbohydrates back into the meal plan. The Atkins diet restricts carbohydrates throughout the entire diet.

While both diets focus on low carbohydrates, the Atkins diet has you actually counting carbohydrates. The South Beach diet does not require any actual counting of carbohydrates.

While both diets can cause ketosis, the Atkins diet actually wants you to put your body into ketosis.

Another difference between the two diets is the amount of phases that the diet has. The South Beach diet is broken into 3 phases while the Atkins diet is broken into 4 phases.

Chapter 8 – The Stillman Diet

The Stillman diet was created by doctor Irwin Maxwell Stillman. This diet is very restrictive in that it cuts out carbohydrates and fats. The focus of the diet seems to center around high protein and nothing else. The diet does offer up some dairy choices that you may choose from. The diet is not restrictive in the amounts of foods that you can eat. In fact you may eat all you want of the foods allowed. The diet is restrictive in that it cuts out almost all forms of food.

With the Stillman diet you are giving 5 areas of foods that you are allowed to eat out of. Lean meats such as beef, lamb and veal are allowed. You can cook these by either broiling, boiling, baking or smoking them. Chicken and Turkey are allowed as well. When preparing these you can either roast, broil or boil the meat. Lean fish and seafood is allowed on the Stillman diet. You may use cocktail sauce, horseradish or ketchup with the fish or seafood. Eggs are allowed to be eaten. You may cook these either by hard boiling, soft or medium boiled, poached or fried but hard boiled is the preferred method for eggs. For dairy you are allowed cottage cheese, farmer cheese and pot cheese that is made from skim milk only. Your are not allowed to use butter, margarine, oil or grease to prepare any of your foods.

For drinking on this diet you must consume 8, 10 ounce glasses of water each day. In addition to you water you are allowed to drink coffee, tea and any carbonated beverage that does not have calories.

Chapter 9 – Pros and Cons of the Stillman Diet

Everything has pros and cons and the Stillman diet is no different. Before deciding on a dieting plan to help you lose weight you must first look at the pros and cons of a the dieting plan. This way you can see both side of the fence and then make an informed decision based on your individual needs and lifestyle.

The pros of the Stillman diet:

- Promotes the consumption of lots of meat. This in itself will appeal to men and thus get them to diet.

- Allows for the drinking of coffee and tea.
- Can aid you in shedding lots of weight in a short amount of time.
- No fruits or vegetables on this diet, so it fits for anyone who already despises fruits and vegetables.
- No counting of calories, fat grams or carbohydrates. Absolutely no counting of anything at all.
- You can eat as much as you want from any of the approved foods.
- The Stillman diet is a high protein diet. Protein is used to build and repair tissue as well as being on the bodies main building blocks for bones, muscles, cartilage, skin and even blood.
- The body does not store protein, therefore a high protein diet keeps you in a steady supply of protein.

From a lot of angles the Stillman diet sounds good. But when looking at the cons of the Stillman diet, some may wonder if it really is all that good after all. It is an individuals decision based on the weighting of both the pros and cons though as to whether this diet is right.

The cons of the Stillman diet:

- Very restrictive food list. Almost no dairy except for three choices, no fruit of any kind, no vegetables of any kind and nothing with fats or carbohydrates.
- Very restrictive way to prepare foods as you can not use any oils, butter, margarine or grease when cooking.

- Extremely high protein diets can be very unhealthy for the heart and other organs.
- Lack of fats and carbohydrates can send the body into ketosis. Ketosis can cause strain on the kidneys. Research is yet to determine what the long term damages are from ketosis.
- Calcium levels are negatively effected on the Stillman diet.
- Complications such as constipation and dehydration can occur while on the Stillman diet, despite how much water it has you drinking.
- Rare complications such as an increase risk of heart disease, hypertension and liver and kidney trouble can happen on the Stillman diet since it cuts out all fat and carbohydrates but allows for a large consumption of protein.

Chapter 10 – Comparing the Stillman Diet and the Atkins Diet

The Stillman diet is closer to the Atkins diet than the South Beach diet is. The South Beach diet works on the bases of eating the right types of carbohydrates. Where as the Stillman diet and the Atkins diet focus on no carbohydrates to low carbohydrates. As well both the Stillman diet and the Atkins diet are high protein diets. In this they both promote the consumption of high amounts of protein. Both believe that the restriction of carbohydrates and the increase in protein will aid rapid weight loss. Both diets are right in their belief that this will allow for rapid weight loss.

The problem is with both of these diets they also come with some potential health risks. Critics point out that both the Stillman diet and the Atkins diet cause ketosis. Ketosis puts a strain on the kidneys and no research can show yet what the long term health risks are. Both diets are also known to increase the risk of heart disease since they promote such high amounts of protein.

While the Stillman diet cuts out all forms of carbohydrates and fats and puts the dieter on a very strict food list, the Atkins diet allows for small amounts of carbohydrates and an unrestricted amount of fats. Most people will use the Stillman diet in connection with the Atkins diet for this reason. While on the Atkins diet some dieters will switch to the Stillman diet to get over any stalls with their weight loss while on the Atkins diet.

It is no wonder that with the similarities in the diets that the Stillman diet was competition for the Atkins diet back in the 1970s. Nor is it any wonder that in today's fad diet era of low carbohydrates that both are making a come back.

Chapter 11 – The Zone Diet

The Zone diet focuses on insulin levels when it comes to weight loss. With the Zone diet the purpose is to obtain the right insulin level that the body needs to have to loss weight and prevent the regaining of the weight back. To obtain the right insulin level when eating a person must have the right ratio of protein to carbohydrates to fat. The ratio that the Zone diet uses is 40 percent protein, 30 percent carbohydrates and 30 percent fat.

The Zone was published in 1995 by Barry Sears, PhD. He has published other books since then that focus on the Zone diet. His official website offers up books written on the Zone, recipes, a FAQ page and also gives explanations of food blocks, carbohydrates and how the Zone is intended to work at losing weight and maintaining weight loss.

The Zone diet breaks these down into individual blocks. Each protein is a block as is each carbohydrate and each fat is a block. For an individual block protein is 7 grams, carbohydrates are 9 grams and fat is 3 grams. The three blocks go together when eating to make what the Zone diet considers to be a complete block. It is when one eats a complete block that insulin levels are at their prime for weight loss. It is then that you have to have so many complete blocks at meal time to achieve the right insulin levels.

The Zone diet allows for the eating of most foods as long as you stick to the 40/30/30 rule of the diet. The official website for the Zone diet has really made it easy to figure out how to eat while on the zone diet. You will of course be using your hand as a guide when doing this. According to the official website for the Zone the normal protein serving will fit into the palm of your hand. So what you do is use a plate that has three sections. One section of course is a little bigger and the other two are to be the same size. These help until you get use to what you are doing when trying to measure out your food. Place your hand sized amount of protein food in the big section then fill the other two with fruit in one and vegetables in the other. Make sure to a small amount of mono-sodium fat to part of your food. Olive oil will work great for this.

Chapter 12 – Pros and Cons of the Zone Diet

Everything has pros and cons and the Zone diet is no different. Before deciding on a dieting plan to help you lose weight you must first look at the pros and cons of a the dieting plan. This way you can see both side of the fence and then make an informed decision based on your individual needs and lifestyle.

The pros of the Zone diet:

- With the zone diet there is never a point where you give up carbohydrates completely or restrict them to very low amounts.

- With the amounts you carbohydrates that you allowed with the Zone you are not putting yourself at risk of going into ketosis.
- With the insulin levels that you will have on the Zone diet you will achieve a sense of fullness. The ability to feel full while on a diet makes it possible for a dieter not to cheat.
- The Zone is viewed by a lot of athletes a perfect diet to help improve their athletic performance.
- As long as you keep with the ratios set up by the Zone diet you can eat out at restaurants.
- Energy levels improve while on the Zone diet for many dieters. This is mostly due to the fact that the Zone diet is designed to normalize insulin levels. When these levels are normalized a person will feel more energetic.

- No counting of Calories while on the Zone diet.
- Another high protein diet that will appeal to men. Thus making it easier to get a man who is in need of a diet on one.

The cons of the Zone diet:

- The Zone diet books are restrictive and can be confusing to a dieter. This makes it hard to follow the diet with a little more clarity being shed on what Barry Sears, PhD meant.
- While you will not have to count calories while on the Zone diet, you will have to count protein grams, carbohydrates and fat grams every time you eat.

- The high levels of protein consumed may put you at risk of heart disease.
- While many athletes believe that the Zone diet helps with performance, not all believe this. Some athletes believe that the amount of carbohydrates allowed on the Zone diet is not enough to prevent muscle cramps and hinder endurance when training.
- There is hardly any research that the claims made that the 40/30/30 ratio is best for normalizing insulin levels.

Chapter 13 – Scarsdale Diet

The Scarsdale diet is an extremely restrictive low calorie diet. This diet has been around since 1979 when it was created by Dr. Herman Tarnower and is considered to be an all or nothing type of diet. Basically with this diet you follow it to the letter or not at all. This diet pushes for no room for any slip ups with it. According to the diet if you do not follow the diet as directed at all times, then the diet will not work at all. Once night eating something you are not supposed to eat will mean that you have to start from square one with the diet again.

With the Scarsdale diet you will only stay on the program for two weeks. Then you will go to the Staying Trim program and then alternate back to the original program. So every two weeks you will alternate between the two programs within the Scarsdale diet.

With the diet you can only eat what foods are on the meal plan set up. All alcohol must be given up while on the diet. Drinks include water, club soda, coffee, tea and any sugar free drinks. When eating a salad you can only use lemon and vinegar or the Scarsdale approved salad dressings. Meat is to be lean meat only and vegetables are to be eaten plain with no butter or anything on them. With the Scarsdale diet no substitutions are allowed at all.

During the two weeks of strict dieting you all pastas, sugar, bread and even potatoes are not allowed at all. While bread is not allowed you may consume high protein bread only. Snacking between meals is also restricted to only carrots or celery. Nothing else is allowed for snacks. The percentages in the diet consist of consuming 43 percent protein with fats reduced down to 23 percent.

The Staying Trim section of the diet is not as restrictive. You will be allowed more foods choices during this time. The amount of protein that you are to consume is also reduced during this phase of the diet.

You must consume plenty of water while on this diet. Without the consumption of a lot of water, you run the risk of kidney failure. So when choosing to follow the Scarsdale diet you must be committed to drinking a lot of water. The reason for this is the build of ketones that are harmful in large quantities in the body. Even during the less restrictive Staying Trim part of the diet, these ketones may still be at high levels in the body.

Another concern with the Scarsdale diet is that it promotes the use of herbal hunger suppressants as well as the use of artificial sweeteners. Increasingly, these suppressants and artificial sweeteners are being linked with a wide assortment of health problems and organ damage.

Chapter 14 – The Pros and Cons of the Scarsdale Diet

The Scarsdale diet does have some pros to it despite how much negative light has been shed onto this diet. The pros and cons of any diet must be weighted before making a decision. Do the benefits of this diet out weight the risks associated with the Scarsdale diet? It is up to each individual to weight these pros and cons against what they are wanting and what they are willing to do to achieve their goals.

The pros of the Scarsdale diet:

- Even though the Scarsdale diet is a low calorie diet, it does not require you to count any calories.The Scarsdale diet is also a low carbohydrate diet but again you don't have to count carbohydrates either.
- There is no limit on portion sizes as long as you only eat what is allowed.
- On the Scarsdale diet you can rapidly loss weight without the feeling of being hungry.
- The extremely restrictive phase is only for a short two week period at a time.
- While caffeine is limited you can still have caffeine though.

The cons of the Scarsdale diet:

- It is an extremely restrictive food plan. This makes it hard for dieters to stick with the diet.
- The Scarsdale diet does not give for any mistakes. If a dieter eats even on thing that is not on the food plan, then the dieter must start all over again.
- This diet is not very restaurant friendly which can make eating out hard.
- The Scarsdale diet switches from a restrictive phase to a less restrictive phase every two weeks. This can cause for some confusion while dieting.
- The Scarsdale diet has extremely low carbohydrate levels. This can send a body into ketosis.

- Dangerous levels of ketones have been known to build up in the body while on the Scarsdale diet.
- The diet promotes the use of herbal hunger suppressants. These are dangerous and have been known to cause death when taken in large amounts.
- The diet promotes the use of artificial sweeteners which have been linked to a wide variety of health problems.
- Large amounts of water must be consumed while on the diet or kidney failure can occur.

Chapter 15 – Comparing the Scarsdale Diet and the Zone Diet

The Zone diet and the Scarsdale diet have some similarities to them. But at the same time they also differ in the way that the diets work. When finding diets that are similar to each other it is important to look at their similarities as well as how they differ from each other before making a decision on which diet to go with.

Similarities between the Zone diet and the Scarsdale diet:

The Zone diet and the Scarsdale diet both use percentages.

Both diets allow you to achieve a sense of fullness. No point will you be left feeling hungry while on either of these diets.

Both diets allow for carbohydrates while on the diet.

Both of these diets boost rapid weight loss in short amounts of time.

Both diets are restrictive and can confuse dieters who are trying to stick with the diet.

Differences between the Zone diet and the Scarsdale diet:

The Zone diet focuses on the 40/30/30 rule of percentages and requires that dieters weigh out the percentages. The Scarsdale diet has percentages focused on protein and fats but do not require that dieters weigh anything since the restrictive food plans do this for you.

While both diets do allow for carbohydrates, they differ in this as well. The Zone diet allows for enough carbohydrates to prevent ketosis. The Scarsdale diet allows for carbohydrates but the amounts allowed are dangerously low.

Both diets can confuse dieters. But even this differs between the two diets. The Zone is confusing because of all the blocks and percentages that are thrown together making a dieter have to figure out how this all works. The Scarsdale diet gets confusing because you switch back and forth between two phases every two weeks.

The Zone diet allows for you to eat almost any food group as long as you keep within the percentages. The Scarsdale diet only allows you to eat a very restrictive set of foods.

The Zone diet gives you enough of what you need to prevent kidney failure. The Scarsdale diet can cause kidney failure if a dieter does not drink enough water.

While on the Scarsdale diet there is not counting of anything. The Zone diet on the other hand has you counting protein grams, carbohydrate grams and fat grams every single time you eat.

Snacks on the Zone diet can consist on anything as long as you keep the percentages right. The Scarsdale diet only allows carrots and celery for snacks.

When eating out at a restaurant the Zone diet is restaurant friendly. The Scarsdale diet is not exactly restaurant friendly since you can only eat certain foods.

Chapter 16 – Health Risks You Run With The Above 5 Diets

Diets have many names are created by different people. But a lot of diets have things in common with them. Some times the similarities are how the diet works and the types of foods allowed. Other times it is the dangers that each diet can pose to the dieter. The dangers involved in any type of diet, should ultimately be looked at. Many times a dieter will be desperate in their attempt to lose weight quickly that they do not take the time to see how many dangers are involved with a particular diet plan. The South Beach diet, Atkins diet, Stillman diet, Zone diet and the Scarsdale diet all pose potential dangers to the dieter.

Ketosis is dangerous as it puts strain on the kidneys. There is little research to show what the long term risks associated with ketosis is. The South Beach diet can cause ketosis during the initial two week phase due to the complete removal of carbohydrates. The Atkins diet actually promotes going into ketosis and restricts your carbohydrates to low levels throughout the diet. With no carbohydrates being allowed at all in the Stillman diet ketosis occurs. The Scarsdale diet also has low carbohydrate levels that cause ketosis.

Out of the above fad diets, the Zone is the only one that does not cause nor promotes ketosis.

Heart diseases are a risk with all of the above fad diets due to their promoting large amounts of animal protein consumption.

These large amounts can clog arteries up rather quickly.

Calcium levels are affected with high protein-low carbohydrate diets. Most of these diets restrict much needed vitamins and minerals that the body needs to stay healthy. The Stillman diet restricts a dieter to no vegetables or fruit. The Scarsdale diet also restricts a lot of foods and can cause calcium levels to drop.

Dehydration and constipation are also caused by all diets that promote high levels of protein and low levels of carbohydrates. When foods are restrictive you are also not getting water from certain foods that you normally would get, therefore you must drink more water to counter dehydration and constipation.

The promotion of herbal suppressants can be dangerous. Herbal hunger suppressants can cause death when taken in large amounts. The negative effects of herbal hunger suppressants are intensified with the consumption of caffeine.

Cholesterol levels may rise once your weight has stabilized with high protein- low carbohydrate diets. High levels of cholesterol can cause health complications.

Chapter 17 –
The Grapefruit Diet

The grapefruit diet is supposed to burn fat away. This diet promotes the grapefruit as the ultimate fat burner. But unlike the images that the name gives you, the grapefruit diet actually consists of eating more foods that just grapefruit. The key though is to eat some grape fruit with each meal. This diet is intended for 12 days straight then a 2 day break before going onto the diet again for 12 days.

The diet has a semi strict 7 day meal plan that gained fame in the 1970s. The restrictions are just that you must eat what you are told, but the amounts that you eat are almost unlimited. The only limit you have on amounts that you can not decrease or increase is the amount of grapefruit that you eat or the amount of the grapefruit juice that you have to eat. As well even though you can eat unlimited amounts you must eat only the foods you are told to eat at each meal.

The following is the minimums that you must eat along with what meal you are to eat them at.

For breakfast you need to consume

½ grapefruit or 8 oz grapefruit juice.

2 eggs prepared any way that you want and 2 slices of bacon.

For lunch you need to consume

½ grapefruit or 8 oz grapefruit juice.

A salad and any form of meat that you want.

For Dinner you need to consume

½ grapefruit or 8 oz grapefruit juice.

You can have either a salad or any red or green vegetable that you want, as well as any type of meat that you want.

You also need to drink 1 cup of coffee or tea with dinner. A bedtime snack is 8 oz of either tomato juice or skim milk.

You may use any type of salad dressing that you want with your salads. All vegetables can be cooked in butter if you wish. Meats can be prepared any way that you want them too. This allows for you to switch things up a little bit each day that you are on the diet.

The above portions are the minimum that you must consume. Make sure at breakfast though that you eat the bacon. The only portions again that you can not change are the grapefruit or the grapefruit juice. It is recommended though that coffee is kept to only 1 cup at dinner. The reason is that the diet believes that coffee will effect insulin levels and thus affect the fat burning process.

With the grapefruit diet you are not allowed to have desserts, breads or any type of white vegetable and even sweet potatoes are not permitted. Other than that you are free to eat vegetables and meats until you are full. The diet seems to play on the side of the more you eat the more fat you will burn.

Chapter 18 – The Pros and Cons of the Grapefruit Diet

The Grapefruit diet has some potentially good points to it. But at the same time it does pose some negative aspects as well. Weight the pros and cons of the Grapefruit diet when determining if this diet is meant for you. Your decision should come from whether or not this diet will fit with your lifestyle and if the cons are worth it taking on or not.

The pros of the Grapefruit diet:

- There are no limits on the amount of foods you can consume from the foods the diet gives you.
- The diet allows for the use of butter on your foods.
- The way you prepare you foods is totally up to you. No restrictions on

the way you prepare you eggs, meat and vegetables.

- You can use any type of salad dressing that you want on your salads.
- No form of meat is restricted during this diet.
- No risk of ketosis since the foods you are allowed to have can contain carbohydrates.
- This diet is actually restaurant friendly, so you can eat out while on this diet.
- No restriction on the way you prepare you food allows for adding variety to the diet.
- Very few foods are restricted while on this diet.
- The structure of the diet is semi relaxed compared to other diets.

The cons of the Grapefruit diet:

- You must eat a grapefruit or drink grapefruit juice with every meal.
- There are no between meal snacking at all while on this diet. The only snack you get is a bedtime liquid snack.
- The freedom to eat virtually anything you want may not allow for a dieter to truly stick to the diet.
- A two day break from the diet may make it hard to go back onto the diet for another 12 days.
- The grapefruit diet is based on the fact that the grapefruit is a fat burner. There is no research that supports this theory.
- Grapefruits can restrict the way the body breaks down certain medications. This can lead to a dangerous level of medication buildup

in the body. So it is not a healthy choice while taking medication.

Chapter 19 –

The Cabbage Soup Diet

The Cabbage Soup diet allows for the consumption of more than just cabbage soup. The idea behind it though is that by consuming this soup you can burn fat away. While there are other foods allowed with the Cabbage Soup diet, this diet is still extremely restrictive.

During the Cabbage Soup diet you will eat the soup every day but what else you are allowed to have is varied from day to day. You will get a varied of foods on this diet but the day meal plans are extremely restrictive.

One day one you will consume fruit along with your soup only. Also while you can eat as much fruit as you want, you can not have bananas at all. To drink on day one you are allowed to have unsweetened teas and cranberry juice along with your water.

Day two allows for you to consume vegetables along with your soup. You can not have peas or corn during day two. Also you are not allowed to eat any fruit on this day. For dinner you can have a baked potato with butter. To drink on day two you can drink unsweetened teas along with water.

Day three allows you to combine day ones foods with day twos foods along with your soup.

Day four you can eat bananas and drink skim milk along with consuming your soup. Nothing else is allowed on this day. You can only eat up to eight bananas on this day though.

Day five you can consume up to 20 ounces of beef or you can substitute the beef for broiled chicken breasts without the skins. Also you can eat up to six fresh tomatoes. You must still eat your soup at least once during day five. Nothing else is allowed this day. Unsweetened teas along with water can be drunk on this day.

Day six you can consume all the beef that you want. Steaks can be eaten up to three. You may have all the vegetables you want, except for the baked potato. You also need to eat your soup at least once during this day as well. Unsweetened teas along with water are allowed on day six.

Day seven you can consume brown rice and vegetables. You may drink as much as you want of unsweetened fruit juice on day seven. You must still consume your soup at least once on this day. Make sure that you are still drinking water.

How to make the cabbage soup:

6 large green onions

2 green peppers

1-2 cans of diced tomatoes

1 bunch of fresh celery

1 packet of Onion Soup Mix

2 cubes of bullion

1 head of cabbage

Cut all the ingredients up and cover with water to cook. Bring to a boil and allow to boil for at least 10 minutes. Then simmer until vegetables are tender. You may add V-8 juice to the mixture. To season you can use salt, pepper or any other spices that you want.

Chapter 20 – Pros and Cons of the Cabbage Soup Diet

The Cabbage Soup diet has some potentially good points to it. But at the same time it does pose some negative aspects as well. Weight the pros and cons of the Cabbage Soup diet when determining if this diet is meant for you. Your decision should come from whether or not this diet will fit with your lifestyle and if the cons are worth it taking on or not.

Pros of the Cabbage Soup diet:

- Can be effective in weight loss when followed strictly for the 7 days you are to be on the diet.

- Can help lay the ground work for the consumption of healthier foods for a junk food addict.
- Allows for the consumption of much needed fruits, vegetables and lean meats. As well as finally allowing brown rice.
- The foods allowed for this diet are fairly inexpensive, so there are no major expenses when going on this diet.
- You are allowed to eat until you are full, therefore there is no real incidence or feeling of hunger while on this diet.

The cons of the Cabbage Soup diet:

- Some dieters suffer from feeling so of weakness while on the diet. As well as suffering from symptoms of headaches.
- Calorie consumption is low on this diet as well as much needed nutrients that a person needs. It is for this reason that some dieters experience the problems listed above.
- Weight gain is common after the 7 days of the diet is up. Thus causing an unwanted weight yo-yo effect while dieting.
- It is hard to prepare such a restrictive diet for yourself if you must still prepare normal meals for the rest of your family.

- A very restrictive daily eating plan, which means a lot of dieters will end up cheating while on this diet even though it is only for seven days.

Chapter 21 – Comparing the Grapefruit Diet and the Cabbage Soup Diet

There are points that should be considered with the Cabbage Soup diet and the Grapefruit diet. While both are different they also have similarities that may or may not be noticeable but are there. So which one should you choice to go on? Well first you should read the pros and cons of both types of diets. As well as taking a close look at what is said about both diets.

Both the Cabbage soup diet and the Grapefruit diet are similar in the fact that they both promote a main ingredient that is suppose to be a metrical food that helps to burn fat. In one diet it is grapefruits and in the other diet it is the famous cabbage soup.

Both diets limit the amount of calories that you will be getting to what is considered to be unhealthy levels. These unhealthy levels can cause some symptoms of illness.

Both diets will allow you to eat as much as you want from their food plans. Thus keeping hunger at bay while on the diet. But the restrictive food plans designed for with each meal or each day on the diet can cause for some dieters to break the rules of the diet.

Both diets cut out what you need to maintain the right amount of vitamins and minerals in the way that they are designed.

Experts attribute the weight loss that dieters have while on the diet to the low amount of calories that you are getting. They discount that the cabbage soup or even the grapefruit is responsible for the weight loss.

Both diets can be used to kick start losing weight but neither is recommended by experts as a long term solution to losing weight. Nor do they suggest staying on the diet for more than one week due to the lack of much needed vitamins and minerals that the diet lacks.

Chapter 22 –The Dangers of Liquid Diets

Liquid diets are making the rounds again in the dieting industry. Liquids diets such as the Lemonade diet and the Green Tea diet are dangerous and can prove very harmful to the body. These diets restrict the amount of solid foods that a person consumes and does not offer up any of the nutrients that the person loses when giving up solid foods.

Both of these liquid diets are more of a fast than a diet. They are geared to replace normal meals with just the drink instead. This causes the body to go into a fasting mode. Ketosis occurs, calcium levels drop, protein levels drop and a dieter may also suffer ill symptoms from calorie reductions, thus putting a person at risk of a variety of health problems.

Ketosis puts strain on the kidneys and there is still very little known about the long term effects of ketosis. As well low calcium levels can lead to problems with the bones, deterioration of the teeth and loss of muscle mass. Protein is need to aid in tissue repair, keeping the blood healthy and it also effects bones and muscle strength. Multiple health problems can occur from low amounts of protein. The body does not store protein therefore protein must be replaced and a liquid diet such as lemonade and green teas does not allow for this. Low amounts of calories can lead to an over all ill feeling as well as cause headaches.

Lemonade or green tea should never be used to replace a meal. It is better to eat a sensible meal and use one of these liquid diets to curb some in between meals snacking. You body needs food for energy, therefore solid foods will help you maintain energy. The more energy you have the more active you will be. Being active will help more to burn fat than anything else. It is not harmful to use green tea or the lemonade recipe that the lemonade diet gives, with your meals. Just do not skip eating and drink just the liquid.

Chapter – 23 Exercise and Fad Diets

Most fad diets do not promote healthy exercising. The ones that do seem to promote it also restrict foods to the point that a dieter is left feeling to tired to exercise. The problem with low carbohydrate diets and exercise is that the body needs carbohydrates in a certain amount to aid in energy and endurance and these low carbohydrate diets usually do not give the needed amount. Carbohydrates not only help with energy and endurance but they also protect muscles from cramping up during physical activities. Muscle cramps can hinder your ability to stay physically active enough for healthy weight loss.

When trying to loss weight one needs to be physically active in order to not only loss the weight but to keep it off. If you rely on a diet to help you drop the weight then go off the diet you will be back to gaining weight. If you use proper exercise and get physically fit you are able to keep the weight off even when you go off the diet.

It is the lack of physical activity that allows for a lot of dieters to fail. When they go off the diet they gain weight back. Some go off the diet because they lost the desired amount of weight. Others go off the diet because it is too restrictive. Either reason the dieter is left even more frustrated when they start to gain the weight back. A dieter can counter all of this by getting up and getting active.

Depression is one of the problems associated with failed dieting and the yo-yo weight gaining and losing. To counter this one should get active. For some they are severely out of shape so it is hard to get physically active. The best way to start is to go out side and walk around in your yard. Just being up and walking is physical activity and can greatly help build you up. Being outside in the sunshine will counter the depression and help to lift your mood and keep you motivated. Then progress to walking around the block. Start small and work your way up. This way when you lose weight you are more likely to keep it off.

With activity being needed, you should look for diets that will not hinder your energy levels. Instead you should look for a dieting plan that gives you all the needed levels of protein, carbohydrates, fats, vitamins and minerals.

Personally, all I did when I realized I had put on a few extra pounds, was walk, for a year, I'd walk around 6 to 8 kilometers per day. I didn't change my diet much, just the amount. (I still enjoy bacon, ice cream, cookies, chocolates etc), granted, currently, I don't have the "six pack" abs, that's just a little more effort. But needless to say, I lost the bulk and got back into the old pants I used to fit into. An unfortunate incident, a back injury, halted my walking at the year and a quarter mark, so instead, I rode a bicycle which put less strain on my back. Just keep active, if you eat more, do more to burn it off. If you don't do much, gauge your eating, eat less in those times. Once again, from a personal perspective, Fad Diets, trendy diets....Stay away from them, just because celebrities, or even your neighbors, friends or associates get on these things doesn't mean you should. A question comes to mind "..who is more foolish, the fool, or the fool that follows.?.."

Chapter 24:

Three Ways to Recognize a Fad Diet

Fad diets have been around for a very long time. Old fad diets are reappearing as revised, with new competition starting up to get in on the diet millions. After all overweight dieters will try anything to lose weight and do so quickly. Even though a person may say that they will not try a fad diet, there are just as many people that will. This keeps the fad diet industry going. The problem with these fad diets is that they are not designed to give lasting results. Therefore you spend the money and the time on the fad diet only to regain the weight. So, generally, one of two things can happen. One, you give up completely on the whole diet thing and write it off as a bad diet and move on to a new dieting plan. Or, two, you start back up on the same fad diet thinking that the weight gain was your fault some how. Well the last scenario is what the makers of that fad diet are hoping for.

The American Heart association had released some ways for dieters to recognize a fad diet so that they may be able to avoid the problems with fad diets. Recognizing a fad diet is easy when one takes the time to look at the warning signs that the American Heart association had released, for example.

Does the diet plan tell you that you can lose a lot of weight in a short amount of time? If so then it would fall under a fad diet. Rapid weight loss is not from losing fat, it is from losing water weight. It is not an ideal solution for dieters to try and loss weight quickly.

Does the diet plan restrict food groups? By restricting food groups dieters are more likely to break the rules of the diet. Restrictive diets do not allow for dieting success. Thus making this a fad diet. After all most fads in any section of life never last for long before they are replaced by a new fad.

Does the diet brag about weight loss with out too much emphasis being put on the exercise? Most health doctors will tell you that it is impossible to truly loss weight and keep the weight off without exercise. There for when a diet brags about weight loss with hardly any emphasis being placed on weight loss then this is another fad diet.

Chapter 25 – "Diet" Soft Drinks and losing weight

As alarm bells rang all over the world regarding the seemingly unstoppable growth in the number of overweight and obese people, men and women the world over, have started to pay more attention to what it is they're eating during an average day. The business sector has also decided to help this new movement toward food and weight awareness by launching series of products that are either fat free or sugar free. The soft drinks producers, for instance, who have taken a lot of flak over the years for selling sugar water, have presented consumers with "diet" or "light" versions of their products.

Diet Coke for example is the Coca-Cola Company's answer to the newly discovered focus on a healthier lifestyle that tries to shun the traditional noon meal of hamburgers and regular Coke. Since many people are trying to avoid the huge amount of unnecessary calories contained in burgers and Coke, they have been offered a healthier choice in the shape of the same soft drink they like, but without the calorie-rich sugar. The success of Diet Coke has proved that customers are interested in healthier alternatives when these become available and that means that fighting obesity at international level may not be as hard as once thought.

Another possible good thing, yet questionable (every report that comes out says something different), about Diet Coke is the presence of caffeine. Some experienced dieters are aware that many weight loss supplements and other kinds of diet pills on the market contain caffeine because this substance has certain desirable effects on the human body. For one thing, caffeine provides extra energy and acts as a stimulant. But that's not all, since caffeine also has a mild appetite suppressant effect. Given that most adults drink caffeine in one form or another anyway, you can use Diet Coke to help stick to your diet and not make things harder for yourself by drinking non-diet soft drinks.

Nevertheless, you should keep in mind the fact that over consumption of any substance is not a good idea so don't drink Diet Coke by the gallon just because it doesn't interfere with your dieting. Prolonged overuse of caffeine can lead to other problems, including ulcer, sleep disorder and anxiety. Trading bad eating habits for a bad Diet Coke habit is plain silly, all things in moderation.

Drinking Diet Coke instead of regular Coke

or other brands of sugar water is a very good idea, IF, there are no suitable alternatives, and you're trying to lose weight. But remember that avoiding sources of unnecessary calories is only part of the greater effort. Keep an eye on the food intake and exercise at least thirty minutes, five times per week. This is the healthy lifestyle that one should strive for, little by little. Don't force yourself thin or healthy all at once.

Chapter 26 – Often Overlooked Diets

There are many different diets out there and they become just that, something you eat on a regular basis. Some are recommended, some followed as in the context of Fad Diets, others which are there but completely overlooked.

You might get bored with the same old thing, habitually, and it might seem that eating healthy is a laborious chore. The truth is it is no different, it just means when you go shopping, you pick alternative products to the saturated fats etc.

And there's nothing to say that you can't do a world tour of "Healthy Dieting", which could become a whole New "Fad" well...the term "Movement", would be preferred something longer lasting more enjoyable different and cultural. It takes approximately 6 weeks to get climatized to your diet, that is for your food to go through your body and you to become your surroundings figuratively speaking. So you can do the whole "Perpetual Global Traveller Diet" in the comfort of your own home. Choose a country and their healthy foods, and cook like that for 3 months, then pick another and do the same and another and so on and so forth. The time for each can vary, that's what makes it unique, I suppose you could call it exciting, but definitely different. You've got a whole world to choose from. And getting the ingredients locally will probably save you an upset stomach in some cases.

Some cultures have their diets linked to their religious beliefs, I`m not saying in these cases to go join any specific belief system, as Food is for Everyone, regardless of personal belief.

For example, the belief in Ayurveda is that 'We are what we eat', a common enough term as you hear it everywhere, so, the Ayurvedic point of view, a good diet is of prime importance. It not only helps to maintain the body's health and vitality, but also has a great effect on the well being of the mind. According to Ayurveda, a truly healthy human being is the one who has a strong body and sound mind.

While it is beyond the scope of this book to go into detail of everything involved, which may be available in other publications, I can briefly mention that they believe a well balanced and nutritious diet helps to maintain the balance of the three doshas and promotes good health. Ayurveda classifies various types of food like vegetables, fruits, nuts, grains, etc on the basis of their energies and the affect that they have on the body and mind. This can help us in choosing the foods that are good for our individual constitution, while avoiding the ones that are likely to be harmful.

Many times, in today's hurried modern lifestyle, irregular eating habits or excessive attachment and consumption of particular foods is common. We often consume more of certain foods which can be harmful for us. Ayurveda suggests what are referred to as 'Antidotes' or balancing factors for such excesses. These balancing factors help to control the negative effects of the food we overeat and can aid in the maintenance of balance in our systems.

Diet is given maximum importance in healthy as well as diseased status. It is said in ancient Indian literature that if proper diet is followed, medicine is not needed, and if proper diet is not observed, medicines are not helpful.

Although diet is an important healing modality in Ayurveda, there are no one-size-fits-all rules. You are unique in your constitutional make-up and your current needs for balance, hence, your dietary needs are unique too. You won't find pre-set body weights by age and gender or calorie counting instructions in ayurvedic dietary theory. What you will find are recommendations to really listen to what your physiology is telling you about what, where, when and how you eat. Food influences not only physical activities, but also psychological activities.

The ayurvedic way of cooking is about bringing together a harmonious collection of fresh wholesome ingredients into a feast for all your senses. In a well-prepared ayurvedic meal, a medley of tastes, textures, colors, aromas and flavors blend together to restore balance to your body, mind, spirit, senses and emotions.

That is just one example, look around keep the diet in focus and don't get to carried away with the rest, but that's a personal choice, you've got a lot to choose from, ayurvedic is Indian, you've got all the other East, West and in between Asian cuisines to explore as well as European, Middle Eastern, and many others.

Where do you start, well, it really doesn't matter, as long as you do. Then just keep going and sooner or later you'll cover most or as many as you want anyway.

Chapter 27 – Fun & Enjoyable Recipes

Flash Roo Roll

- 400grams Kangaroo rump steak (you can use lean beef, lamb, pork, deer, rabbit etc)

- 3 teaspoons Worcestershire sauce

- 2 teaspoons seeded mustard

- 1 medium bunch (about 12 spears) of fresh asparagus.

- 1 red pepper (capsicum, can substitute chilies also depending on your taste, spicy stuff tends to raise the metabolism)

- 2 tablespoons oil

Wrap the kangaroo steak in plastic wrap and freeze for about 20 minutes or until partially frozen. Remove the plastic and cut into thin slices (tenderizing with a meat tenderizer is optional). Combine steak, sauce and mustard in a bowl and cover, then refrigerate for 30 minutes.

Cut the asparagus and pepper into 5cm (2 inch) strips. Boil steam or microwave asparagus and pepper until just tender, then drain. Wrap a piece of steak around a 1 piece of asparagus and 1 piece of pepper and secure with a toothpick. Repeat with the remaining steak, asparagus and pepper.

Just before serving, heat veggie oil in pan add the rolls, cook until well browned all over.

Makes about 48

Rolls can be prepared a day ahead, can be stored in refrigerator, the uncooked rolls can be frozen, not suitable for microwave.

Lamb Kebabs With Herb Yoghurt dip

- Wooden Kebab skewers
- 750g lean lamb (you can try pork, beef etc.)
- 1 onion - grated
- 1 clove garlic - crushed
- 1 teaspoon ground cinnamon
- 2 teaspoons paprika
- 2 teaspoons ground cumin
- 1/4 teaspoon chili powder
- 2 tablespoons chopped fresh mint
- 1/4 cup chopped fresh parsley
- 1 tablespoon dry red wine

Combine lamb, onion, garlic, spices, herbs and wine in a bowl and mix well.

Shape about a tablespoon of mixture around one end of skewers.

Just before serving, grill sticks until well

browned all over and cooked right through.
Serve hot with dip.

Herb Yoghurt Dip

- 500grams plain yoghurt
- 2 cloves garlic, crushed
- 1 tablespoon chopped fresh parsley
- 2 tablespoons chopped fresh mint
- 1 tablespoon chopped fresh chives

Combine all ingredients in a bowl and mix
well.

Makes about 40

Sticks and sauce can be prepared a day
ahead.

Store covered in refrigerator.

Freezing unused sticks is ok, but not
freezing the sauce.

Not suitable for Microwave.

Green Beans Side Dish

- 2 cups chopped green beans
- 2 tablespoon olive oil or ghee
- 2 tsp brown or black mustard seeds
- A few red pepper flakes
- 2 tsp lemon juice
- 1/2 tsp turmeric
- 1 tsp minced ginger
- 1 tsp black pepper
- Rock or sea salt to taste
- 2 tbsp white sesame seeds
- 4 tbsp fresh grated coconut
- 2 tbsp chopped cilantro

Steam the beans for 10 minute. In a non-stick pan, heat the olive oil.

Add the mustard seeds.

As the seeds start popping, add the beans, turmeric, minced ginger, lemon juice, salt, black pepper and red pepper flakes and sauté for a few minutes. Beans should be tender but not mushy. Reduce heat to low.

In another pan, toast the sesame seeds for a few minutes until they turn light brown.

Transfer beans to a serving dish. Top with the sesame seeds, grated coconut and cilantro and serve warm with whole grain bread and lentils.

(Serves 3–4)

Broccoli and Mung Bean Bake

- 1 cup mung beans (split hulled mung beans)
- 2 cups chopped broccoli florets
- 6-8 cups water
- 1-2 tbsp lime juice
- 1 tsp minced fresh ginger
- 2-4 tbsp chopped fresh cilantro
- 4 tbsps cooking oil
- Salt and fresh ground black pepper to taste

Wash the mung beans. Add water and cook until tender. Stir occasionally and remove any foam that forms on top. Drain.
Add the broccoli, lime juice, ginger, salt and black pepper and mix gently

Rub cooking oil on the bottom and sides of a shallow baking dish.

Scoop the mixture into the dish and drizzle the rest of the ghee on top.

Bake at 350-375 degrees for 20 minutes.

Garnish with cilantro and serve warm.
(Serves 2)

Indian Chapatis

- 2 cups whole wheat flour
- 1/3 cup yogurt
- 1⁄2 to 3⁄4 cup water as needed
- ghee or melted butter

In bowl combine flour and yogurt. Gradually add water, mixing with your hands until you have a soft dough. Knead for 5 minutes on floured tabletop.

Divide dough into 12 pieces. Roll each piece into a ball and then press flat in the palms of your hands.

Place a cast iron skillet on medium heat so it will be a little hot by the time you are ready to cook the first chapati.

Roll flattened balls into 5-inch circles on a table or board covered with flour. Try to make the chapati as round as possible. After it is rolled, place on skillet. When the chapati starts bubbling on one side, turn it over and cook on the other side. This takes about 20 seconds on each side.

While first chapati is cooking in skillet, turn second burner on to medium heat. (If you have an electric range, use a small grill over the burner.)

After the chapati has been cooked in skillet, quickly take a pair of tongs and hold the chapati gently over medium heat until it puffs up. This should take about 5 seconds. Then hold chapati with tongs on other side and cook for another 5 seconds. Chapati will look like it is freckled with brown spots. Don't be discouraged if the chapati doesn't puff up all the time. This takes practice.

Brush with melted butter or oil.

GT Beans

Ingredients

- 1 3/4 cups split green peas or whole green beans
- 6 1/2 cups of water
- 1 tablespoon sunflower/veggie oil
- 1/2 teaspoon mustard seeds
- 1/2 teaspoon turmeric
- 1/8 to 1/4 teaspoon asafetida
- 1 teaspoon sea salt
- 1 1/2 teaspoon barley malt or brown rice syrup
- 1 1/2 teaspoon lime or lemon juice
- 1 teaspoon coriander powder
- 1/2 teaspoon cinnamon
- 1/4 teaspoon curry powder, mild
- 1/4 – 1/2 cup red & green pepper, chopped (optional, omit for Pitta)

Preparation Method: Soak green whole beans for 2 hours and then drain. (If using split peas, soak for 1/2 hour)

Heat the oil in a large sauce pan.

Add mustard seeds and when they pop add turmeric, asafetida, green beans, water and rest of the ingredients.

Mix them well.

Cover and cook until beans become quite soft and preparation thickens.

For split green peas it may take 1/2–1 hour and for whole green beans 1 –2 hours.

Quick Tip This tastes good with the chapatis, buttermilk curry, rice and vegetables. The beans can be soaked overnight if convenient. Alternatively it can be garnished with peppers and dry ginger, or other garnishes to suit personal taste.

Herb Rolls

- 2 tablespoons yeast
- 1 1⁄2 cups warm water (105°)
- 1/3 cup buttermilk
- 1 tablespoon sugar
- 1 teaspoons salt
- 1⁄2 cup melted butter
- 3 cups flour
- 1 teaspoon oregano
- 1 1⁄2 teaspoons basil leaves
- 1 tablespoon chopped parsley
- 1⁄4 teaspoon hing

In a large bowl add yeast to water and let sit for 30 seconds.

Add melted butter, spices, buttermilk, salt, and sugar.

Gradually stir bowl with a little butter and add dough. Cover and let rise in warm kitchen area until doubled in bulk (approximately 45 minutes). Fold dough over, punch down, and knead 1 minute.

Preheat oven to 375°. Grease muffin pans. Make 36 small balls about 1-inch each. Fill greased muffin tins with 3 balls each. They will look like a cloverleaf.

Cover and let rise for 1 hour.

Bake for 15 minutes or until golden brown.

Serve hot with butter.

Makes 1 dozen rolls.

Easy Black Beans with Veggies

Ingredients

- 1 tablespoon olive oil
- 1/2 cup chopped celery
- 1/2 cup chopped carrot
- 1/2 cup each seeded and chopped red and green bell pepper
- 4 cups cooked black beans (approximately three and a half cups, raw)
- 2 cups vegetarian stock or water
- 4 teaspoons chili powder, or more to taste
- 1/2 teaspoon oregano
- 1/4 cup chopped cilantro
- 2 tablespoons honey, tomato paste, yogurt, grated monterey jack cheese (for garnishing)

Preparation Method: Heat oil in a large pot and sauté celery, carrot, bell pepper for 5 minutes, stirring frequently.

Add the rest of the ingredients (except garnishing ingredients) and boil.

Lower the heat, cover with the lid and simmer for 45 minutes to 1 hour or till consistency becomes thick.

Remove from heat and garnish with green onion, cheese and a dollop of yogurt.

Mixed Vegetables in Almond Sauce

- 1 cup vegetables of your choice, cut into 1/4" dice (choose from asparagus, carrots, green beans, green peas, parsnips, beets)
- 1 cup mixed tender greens, shredded
- 1 cup stock (beef, chicken etc) , in 1/4" cubes (optional, as is your choice of stock, experiment)
- 2 tsp cumin seed
- 1/2 tsp minced fresh ginger
- 1/4 tsp ground clove
- 1/4 tsp ground cinnamon
- 1/4 tsp ground cardamom
- 1/4 tsp turmeric
- 1/2 tsp fresh-ground black pepper
- Rock salt to taste
- 1/2 cup fresh unflavored yogurt , preferably homemade
- 30–40 almonds, soaked in warm water and blanched
- 8 cups water
- 2 Tbsp veggie oil

- 3 Tbsp finely chopped cilantro

Steam the vegetables for about 7-8 minutes. Grind together the almonds, ginger and yogurt with about half the water to a very smooth puree. Add the water in increments as needed to grind.

Heat the oil in a large pot.
Add the cumin seeds and stir briefly to release flavor and aroma.

Reduce heat to medium and add the greens and the powdered spices. Stir-fry for about 2-3 minutes; then add the rest of the water and bring to a boil.

Fold in the sauce and the steamed vegetables, add salt, reduce heat to low, cover and simmer for about 7-8 minutes, stirring occasionally to prevent burning or sticking.

Add the stock cubes, stir briefly and remove from heat.

Garnish with chopped cilantro and serve hot with plain rice.
(Serves 2–3)

Chapter 28 – A potentially deadly "side effect" of obesity. - Diabetes.

There are many other problems attributed to obesity or just generally being overweight. And the condition is in general and more often than not attributed to a poor Diet, it is of great concern and one of the reasons for including this chapter.

Diabetes is Australia's fastest growing chronic disease. While Type 1 diabetes represents 10-15% of all diabetes, it is the growth in Type 2 diabetes, 85-90% of all cases, which causes particular concern as it relates to lifestyle, over one million Australians have diabetes – 100,000 Australians are developing diabetes each year, and 200,000 people move from overweight to obese.

In just the United States alone, diabetes affects over 16.9 million people or 8.6% of adults (age 20 or over) and costs the nation almost $100 billion each year.

Internationally, the figures for diabetes stricken people are shocking!

Diabetes is a chronic metabolic disease characterized by high glucose (sugar) levels in the blood. Insulin, a hormone produced by the pancreas, regulates the amount of glucose in the blood.

In patients with diabetes, the body either does not produce enough insulin, or does not adequately respond to the insulin it is producing. This causes blood sugar levels to be higher than normal.
Diabetes can be associated with serious complications such as heart disease, blindness, kidney failure, stroke and lower-limb amputations, but steps can be taken to control the disease and lower the risk of complications.

Type 1 diabetes: Type 1 Diabetes (previously called insulin-dependent diabetes mellitus (IDDM) or juvenile-onset diabetes) develops when the body's immune system destroys pancreatic beta cells, which make insulin.

Type 1 diabetes usually occurs in children and young adults, who must have insulin delivered by injections or a pump in order to survive. Type 1 diabetes may account for 5% to 10% of all diagnosed cases of diabetes. Risk factors include autoimmune, genetic, and environmental factors.

Type 2 diabetes: Type 2 diabetes (previously known as non insulin-dependent diabetes mellitus (NIDDM) or adult-onset diabetes) develops gradually, and is usually caused by a combination of impaired secretion of insulin and reduced sensitivity of the body's cells to insulin (insulin resistance). As a result, blood glucose levels become elevated.

Type 2 diabetes usually occurs in adults, however it is increasingly being diagnosed in people at a younger age, even in childhood and adolescence. Type 2 diabetes may account for about 90% to 95% of all diagnosed cases of diabetes, and the prevalence is rising at an alarming rate throughout the world.

This is believed to be due to increases in longevity, sedentary lifestyles and a dramatic upsurge in obesity.

Type 2 diabetes can be controlled. Therapeutic lifestyle management such as following a careful diet and exercise program and losing excess weight may help, though oral medications are often necessary. Risk factors include older age, obesity, and a family history of diabetes, prior history of gestational diabetes, impaired glucose tolerance, physical inactivity, and race/ethnicity.

Indigenous Australians, Indigenous New Zealanders, African Americans, Hispanic/Latino Americans, American Indians, and some Asian Americans and Pacific Islanders are at particularly high risk for type 2 diabetes.

Other types:

Impaired Glucose Tolerance (IGT): Impaired Glucose Tolerance is an intermediate state between normal blood glucose control and type 2 diabetes. IGT is an early sign that a person's carbohydrate metabolism is impaired. It carries a high risk of progressing to type 2 diabetes. IGT (and type 2 diabetes) result from a combination of impaired secretion of insulin and reduced sensitivity of the body's cells to insulin (insulin resistance).

Gestational diabetes: Gestational diabetes is a form of glucose intolerance diagnosed in some women during pregnancy, but usually disappears after the mother gives birth. Treatment is required to normalize blood glucose levels to avoid complications in the infant. Gestational diabetes occurs more frequently among African Americans, Hispanic/Latin Americans, and Native

Americans. It is also more common among obese women and women with a family history of diabetes.

Secondary diabetes: Secondary diabetes can result from other conditions such as specific genetic syndromes, surgery, drugs, malnutrition, infections, and other damage to or diseases of the pancreas.

How Is Diabetes Diagnosed

Type 1: Patients with type 1 diabetes usually develop symptoms over a short period of time, and the condition is often diagnosed in an emergency setting. Urinalysis of an acutely ill type 1 diabetic patient will detect high glucose levels, and high levels of ketones. Ketones are produced by the breakdown of fat and muscle, and they are toxic at high levels. Ketones in the blood cause a condition called "acidosis" (low blood pH). Blood glucose levels are also high.

Type 2: Patients with type 2 diabetes develop symptoms over a longer period of time. Type 2 diabetes is diagnosed when:

The blood glucose is 126 milligrams per deciliter (mg/dl) or higher on two occasions after fasting (abstaining from food) for 8 or more hours; or

The blood glucose level is 200 mg/dl or higher at any time between meals with symptoms of diabetes, such as increased thirst, urination, and fatigue; or A blood glucose level drawn two hours after drinking a 75-gram glucose solution is 200 mg/dl or higher.

Diabetes: Risk Factors and Preventative Measures

Risk factors are characteristics that can predispose you to developing a condition or disease. Just because you have one or more risk factors does not mean you will get diabetes. Risk factors for type 1 diabetes are not as clearly defined as for type 2 diabetes.

Type 1 diabetes risk factors include:
- Family history of diabetes
- Autoimmune disease, where the body mistakenly attacks the insulin-producing cells.
- Environmental factors

Type 2 diabetes risk factors include:
- Age of 45 years or older
- Obesity
- Family history of diabetes

- Diabetes during pregnancy
- Impaired glucose tolerance (IGT)
- Physical inactivity
- Being a Indigenous Australian, New Zealander, Native American, African American, Hispanic/Latino American, Asian American, or a Pacific Islander just to name a few.

Aside from diet there are other aides and methods are available to assist in management of the condition or conditions. There are safe and natural ways to increase your insulin production and regulate your blood glucose levels. Ofcourse, your doctor will put you on prescription drugs and blood testing for the rest of your life but it's never that simple, as the prescription drugs can be just as harmful as the diabetes itself. The toxic side effects of some of the prescription drugs include weight gain, respiratory infections, nausea, and diarrhea, skin rash, liver damage, headaches and that's just naming a few.

As everyone's biochemistry is different it goes pretty much without saying, that what works for one, may not work for another, or just not work as well. That is the case with whatever you try, whether it's prescription drugs or natural alternatives, trading, or mlm programs even, just to name other instances as examples. As I can't tell you what your doctor will give you, I can tell you there are a number of alternatives that are proving to be quite promising, going by people's personal experiences, these are quite the same if not better than lab reports, because of the fact that any given number of people have tried the product, as opposed to rats in a cage, then human trials, then another ten years, then if you're not already dead and buried, you've more than likely forgotten about it, and they've thrown you onto something else.

One of the main constituents of Diabetagon™ Basic, which is just one such alternative, has also been found to show inhibitory activity on Aldose Reductase which is related to such chronic diabetic complications as peripheral neuropathy, retinopathy, and cataracts etc. It naturally increasing your body's own insulin and helps to regulate and improve glucose tolerance. With improved glucose tolerance the body will become more responsive to the presence of glucose in your blood. Lack of sensitivity is a prime indicator of Type 2 diabetes and controlling your body's sensitivity and tolerance will help you keep a firm grip on controlling and/or preventing diabetes.

Chapter 29 – Resources

The following are resources to help you with your dieting endeavors.

The South Beach Diet:

The South Beach Diet by Arthur Agatston

The South Beach Diet Dining Guide by Arthur Agatston

The Atkins Diet:

Dr. Atkins' New Diet Revolution by Dr. Robert Atkins

Dr Atkins' New Diet Cookbook by Dr. Robert Atkins

The Stillman Diet:

The Doctor's Quick Weight Loss Diet by Irwin Stillman

Dr Stillman's 14 Day Shape Up Program by Irwin Stillman

The Zone Diet:

A week in the Zone: A Quick Course in the Healthiest Diet for You by Barry Sears and Deborah Kotz

Zone Perfect Cooking Made Easy by Gloria Bakst and Mary Goodbody

The Scarsdale Diet:

Complete Scarsdale Medical Diet by Herman Tarnower

1. http://astore.amazon.com/fad-diet-20
2. http://healthbuy.com/article/rss/372021
3. http://lifeforce.net/20478074
4. http://lottobusta.com/extremeherbs (Cooking herbs & weight loss sections)

Book buyers special offer

15% OFF listed retail prices. (current @ 2008)

SPECIAL OFFER PRODUCT DESCRIPTIONS

GLUCOSAMINE PLUS - Glucosamine is the structural component of joint cartilage, ligaments, tendons and synovial fluid, which functions to lubricate and cushion joints. Glucosamine Plus is associated with alleviating osteo and rheumatoid arthritic inflammation and stiffness of joints, as well as assist in the speedy recovery from sports and other minor injuries.

Item Code: SWH-6122   Retail $56.65 BkbuyersDisc. $48.15

VITAMIN B COMPLEX - B Vitamins are water soluble, which means that they are not stored in the body, so they are needed on a daily basis. The primary function of B vitamins is to assist in the release of energy from carbohydrates, fats and proteins in the body, and is beneficial in times of stress.

Item Code: SWH-10132 Retail $37.85 BkbuyersDisc. $32.17

GINKGO BILOBA PLUS - Assists in the maintenance of peripheral circulation and in addition, helps to maintain memory function.

Item Code: SWH-202492 Retail $63.95 BkbuyersDisc. $54.35

OMEGA-3 PLUS - Beneficial in maintenance of cell membranes, general wellbeing and helps maintain healthy cholesterol levels.

Item Code: SWH-2127   Retail $44.15 BkbuyersDisc. $37.52

CHOLESTEROL HEALTH - This unique formula assists in controlling LDL cholesterol (bad) and helps maintain a normal LDL/HDL (good) ratio, helping maintain a healthy heart.

Item Code: SWH-100070 Retail $61.25 BkbuyersDisc. $52.06

HEART CARE - Assists in maintaining a healthy heart. Helps reduce the symptoms of colds, flu, catarrh and hay fever. Gives you the option of taking garlic with out the unpleasant odor side effects.

Item Code: SWH-6160   Retail $40.45 BkbuyersDisc. $34.38

EYE FORMULA VISION PLUS - Rich in vision supporting nutrients, and provides a powerful antioxidant action to reduce oxidative damage (aging) in the retina.

Item Code: SWH-202491 Retail $65.45 BkbuyersDisc. $55.63

LIVER HEALTH - Helps protect the liver from free radical damage and aid in its regeneration.

Item Code: SWH-100352 Retail $33.06 BkbuyersDisc. $28.10

MENOPAUSE RELIEF - Helps relieve menopausal symptoms such as hot flushes, night sweats and mood swings. Provides additional nutritional benefits for overall wellbeing.

Item Code: SWH-6190 Retail $57.15 BkbuyersDisc. $48.57

WOMENS HEALTH PRIMROSE PLUS - Helps provide temporary relief from premenstrual symptoms such as abdominal bloating, tenderness, mild anxiety, and irritability.

Item Code: SWH-6108 Retail $68.75 BkbuyersDisc. $58.43

MENS PROSTATE HEALTH - Helps manage BPH, and assists to support and enhance masculine needs and general wellbeing.

Item Code: SWH-202493 Retail $53.55 BkbuyersDisc. $45.50

ECHINACEA - Helps boost immune system.

Item Code: SWH-111 Retail $68.10 BkbuyersDisc. $57.88

ANTISTRESS FORMULA - Assists in relieving tension, mild anxiety and insomnia. Has calming effects.

Item Code: SWH-6167 Retail $48.22 BkbuyersDisc. $40.98

CARB BLOCKER - Reduces the absorption of both simple and complex carbohydrates can assist in weight loss.

Item Code: SWH-100193 Retail $52.31 BkbuyersDisc. $44.45

BETA CAROTENE PLUS - Assists in good night vision, and helps support the immune system. Beta Carotene is converted to vitamin A as and when the body needs it, otherwise it acts as an antioxidant.

Item Code: SWH-2011 Retail $44.61 BkbuyersDisc. $37.91

PARASELENIUM-E - Antioxidant helps reduce oxidation of LDL lipids, and supports a healthy immune system and heart.

Item Code: SWH-3178 Retail $64.75 BkbuyersDisc. $55.03

FRUIT & VEG CONCENTRATE - Equivalent to more than 10 (ten) servings of fruits and vegetables. Helps maintain optimal health and maintain eye health.

Item Code: SWH-102992 Retail $51.15 BkbuyersDisc. $43.47

VITAMIN C - This formula helps fight free radicals, and assists in reducing the severity of symptoms of colds and flu, and assist with relief from symptoms of allergies.

Item Code: SWH-130 Retail $39.50 BkbuyersDisc. $33.57

VITAMIN C CHEWABLES - Contains important nutrient for the development and maintenance of bones, cartilage, teeth and gums in growing children.

Item Code: SWH-6109 Retail $39.95 BkbuyersDisc. $33.95

DAILY MULTIVITAMIN & MINERAL - Helps provide all the nutrients you need daily in a once a day tablet.

Item Code: SWH-123 Retail $33.45 BkbuyersDisc. $28.43

All above prices are in Australian Dollars

Make your selection, fill in the order form on the following page or print it out neatly, and mail with payment. Bank drafts are acceptable, International orders should be drawable on an Australian bank

Fad Dieting Book Special Offer Order Form

Item Code	Description	Price	Quantity	Total

Sub Total	
Australia + 10% GST	
+Postage / Shipping ____ Australia $15 ____International$35	
Total	

Split Whisker Holdings, Contact Management
c/o- 40 Mathoura Street, Midland, W.A. 6056
Australia

Money Orders / Cheques payable to
Split Whisker Holdings

Orders will be sent as soon as payment clears

Delivery Details:

Name:_____

Address:_____

_____.

Suburb:_____

State:_____.

Postal Code/ZIP Code:_____.

Country:_____.

eMail(if any):_____

Tel:_____

Fax(if any):_____

If Paying by Credit Card Enter Payment Details below:

_| MasterCard   _| Visa   _| American Express

Card Number:_____

Name on Card:_____

Expiry Date:(MM/YY)_____/_____ CVV2#_____

Cardholder
Signature:_____

Fad Dieting Book Special Offer Order Form

Item Code	Description	Price	Quantity	Total

Sub Total	
Australia + 10% GST	
+Postage / Shipping ____ Australia $15 ____International$35	
Total	

Split Whisker Holdings, Contact Management
c/o- 40 Mathoura Street, Midland, W.A. 6056
Australia

Money Orders / Cheques payable to
Split Whisker Holdings

Orders will be sent as soon as payment clears

Delivery Details:

Name:_____

Address:_____

_____.

Suburb:_____

State:_____.

Postal Code/ZIP Code:_____.

Country:_____.

eMail(if any):_____

Tel:_____

Fax(if any):_____

If Paying by Credit Card Enter Payment Details below:

_| MasterCard   _| Visa   _| American Express

Card Number:_____

Name on Card:_____

Expiry Date:(MM/YY)_____/_____ CVV2#_____

Cardholder
Signature:_____

Notes:

Notes:

978-0-9805133-0-1

ISBN 978-0-9805133-0-1

9 780980 513301

RRP: $37.95

www.ingramcontent.com/pod-product-compliance
Lightning Source LLC
Chambersburg PA
CBHW072153270326
41930CB00011B/2413